Life is just...

Copyright © 2016 MadeGlobal

ISBN-13: 978-84-944893-4-1

All rights reserved. No part of this publication may be reproduced, stored in a retrieval system, or transmitted, in any form or by any means, electronic, mechanical, photocopying, recording or otherwise, except as permitted by the UK Copyright, Designs and Patents Act 1988, without the prior permission of the publisher.

This is a work of fiction. Names, characters, businesses, places, events and incidents are either the products of the author's imagination or used in a fictitious manner. Any resemblance to actual persons, living or dead, or actual events is purely coincidental.

M
MadeGlobal Publishing

For more information on
MadeGlobal Publishing, visit our website:
www.madeglobal.com

Life is Just One Day

A Collection of Unique Poetry

Suzanne Crossley

"The life of one we love is never lost ......
Its influence goes on through all the lives
it ever touched."

Helen Steiner Rice

A huge thank you goes to the medical team at The Queen Elizabeth hospital Birmingham who treated Suzanne. Our love goes out to the medical teams throughout the world who are trying to find a cure for the devastating T Cell lymphoma illnesses and we hope they may one day find a breakthrough.

The Marshall and Crossley Families

Foreword

In July 2012 at the age of forty I was given the life altering news that I had Cutaneous T Cell Lymphoma . I was at stage 4 of "Sezary Syndrome", an aggressive form of cancer affecting the blood and skin. I was given a twelve-month terminal prognosis and told there was no cure. I was a teacher, a wife and a mother of two sons, and I could also claim I was one in a million, being diagnosed with such a rare illness.

My hair was falling out and I was constantly itching , my feet and hands were cracked so I was struggling to walk and perform basic tasks; I also had to retire from teaching, a job I loved dearly. My life became centred around hospital visits and treatment.

My diagnosis coincided with the establishment of a UK treatment centre at the Queen Elizabeth Hospital, Birmingham, under the guidance of Dr Julia Scarisbrick, a consultant specialising in this rare disease. In 2013, I was offered a bone marrow transplant from an Italian donor - what an amazing person to offer me a chance of more time with my family!

Cancer is a journey with all its ups and downs, it certainly isn't all bad. I feel privileged in a way to have had the diagnosis as it has allowed me to focus on enjoying life, watching my sons mature, listening to the birds, observing the wonder of nature in my garden, sharing a meal, and laughing with my husband and family.

Suzanne Crossley

A personal note

My daughter Suzanne was a very special person whose courage when facing her cancer diagnosis and the pioneering treatments she endured was quite remarkable. With her strength and determination she made the most of everyday and every experience, and never gave up hope.

She had a positive outlook on life but had a true level of understanding of her illness. She was an inspiration to her family and friends. She enriched the lives of everyone who knew her. The world should always be a better place because someone has lived and that is certainly true of my amazing daughter Suzanne.

In July 2015, whilst on the last day of a holiday in Austria, Suzanne suffered a heart attack, lapsed into unconsciousness, and died peacefully with her family by her side.

Janet Marshall (Mother of Suzanne)

Contents

Escape 2
Fear 3
Diagnosis 4
My donor 5
Beauty 6
Hope (I love being alive) 8
Comfort or confined 10
A chance encounter 12
Life is just one day 13
The waiting room 14
A letter to my doctor 15
ABOUT SUZANNE CROSSLEY 17

Escape

Today I'd rather be anywhere else,
Somewhere else, anywhere else
Today I'd rather be anyone else,
Someone else, but me.

I'd take a plane and fly away
To a sunny place, to a peaceful place,
I'd take a plane and soar away
To a space meant just for me.

I'd forget the cancer that soars through my vein
As I wait for a doctor to call my name
I'd forget the cancer that soars through my vein
I'd have my life back you see.

But stop, chin up, I hear myself say
Be strong, be brave for one more day.
Be positive and hope some more
That the cancer will be no more.

So I get up again and face my day,
Put on a smile and hear myself say
Let's go to the hospital just one more time
And believe that the victory can be mine.

Today I'd rather be anywhere else,
Somewhere else, anywhere else
Today I'd rather be anyone else,
Anyone, but me.

29 July 2013

Fear

Fear is such a strange thing
You can't touch it, but you can feel it
You can't see it but you can hear it
You can't take hold of it but it can take hold of you.

It descends with its strong words about the worst that could be
It takes over your thought and mind
Until you can hear nothing else
It chills you to the bone and makes you bow down in
        submission.

But do I have to listen? Do I have to accept it?
How can I drive it away when it seems so powerful.
I simply choose
I turn and whisper 'no'
With faith and love I will not be overwhelmed.

I start to think my quiet thoughts of hope
I think of life and friends
I think of all the good things I can do
I think of all the people I can help,
I think of all the places I can see
I think of all the times I'll have with friends and family.

So I stand, I won't bow down
Fear has fled, its cold hand has gone
The support I receive, the choices I make to live
Drive away this strange thing called fear
This tiny thing called fear.

30 July 2013

Diagnosis

I sit in a stark white room with bright lights
and three doctors who I know will deliver bad news.
They can't meet my eyes,
they look just past me in an attempt
at their own self-preservation.
The bombshell they unleash.
It's cancer stage 4, about as bad as it gets.
I hear them say 12 months to live.
12 months to enjoy, 12 months to live.

I hear their stark words without understanding
I hear their brutal words without comprehending.
I feel nothing inside.

I'm empty, no feeling.
Nothing is out of the ordinary.

So I proceed to take out my question list,
and ask away one by one.
I listen and plan for treatments.
I listen to the list of despicable side effects.
As I leave I look in their eyes and see pity and little hope.
Yet I feel nothing inside, just numbness.

I step outside the room and start to look for the person
that received this news.
I look from the earth to the heavens to search
for this poor person,
who must be hiding and crying somewhere.
So I look some more. I want to help.
But there is no one to see.
I really don't understand.

They can't be, they simply can't be.
They are not talking about me!

30 July 2013

My donor

Somewhere in the world today a kind man, a selfless man
Will go through trial and discomfort just for me.
Somewhere in the world today a nameless man, a humble man
Will give me a second chance to live and be.

A man I have never met, someone's brother, someone's son
Will give up a day for me
A man full of compassion, with the kindest heart
Will give me a chance to live, to be.

Let's raise a toast to this awesome man
Who gives so freely, without self gain
Let's shout from the rooftops for this hero,
This hero without a name.

22 August 2013

Beauty

I read my women's magazines. I look at what they say,
So full of stories and ideas to help us everyday.
I love the articles on fashion, I can already taste the recipes,
I read about how to turn my home into a Mecca of idealism.

As I read on, I start to wonder and question the guides within.
It says how to style my hair, how to look and be thin.
It tells me how to do my nails, with poise and such flair.
It shares the models secrets so no blemish or wrinkle is there.

I turn to my mirror and stare,
My once thick hair, it is fallen out and gone.
My once polished nails are split and ready to shed.
My face is swollen, grotesque from the steroids I must use.
My skin is red and burnt, my feet too sore to walk

People stare when I go out, not with sympathy,
But rubber necking to see this freak, who so offends their sensibility.
Little pity in their eyes- I hear them shout- go away, please hide.
Yet I hold my head up with pride!

You see, I know no matter what people see, that there is a deep beauty in me.
Where the radiotherapy robbed me of my hair,
I have found inner peace
Where cancer has taken my nails, I find incredible strength.
My skin, so red and sore, hides such beauty deep inside.

contd...

So I look into the eyes of others
With a serenity we rarely know,
I sigh and look at my magazine,
How could they get it so wrong?
How could they think its all about show?
Would they follow their own guidelines,
    if this happened to them?
Or would they stop and see the real beauty we all possess.
The beauty devoid of perfection,
Yet, a beauty that can give you life.

2 August 2013

Hope (I love being alive)

I was told some dreadful news,
        awful news,
              the worst that could be.
Failed transplant, lymphoma back,
        no cure.
My world shattered around me as I looked at my bleak future.
Darkness settled over me like a suffocating blanket,
        I can't move,
        I can't get up,
        I can't think.

I have to tell my family, and watch them crumble.
I watch my sweet husband,
        so brave and
        so strong.
As his world falls apart.
What can I do?

Through the fog I hear a small voice:
        Though I walk through the
        valley of the shadow of death
        I will fear no ill, for he is with me.

I sigh and breathe.
The voice speaks again:
        The Lord shall fight for you
        and you shall hold your peace.

I breathe a little easier.
I shall hold on.
I will not give up.
I have hope right in the centre of the darkness,
and I shall cling onto it for dear life as it will see me through.

                                        contd...

Today I was told the news was not correct,
It's too early to tell,
I must trust and wait and believe in hope.
I took refuge under the wings of an eagle,
I was carried through the week by powerful hands that I trusted.
Today I can stop shaking, keep hoping and believing.
I love being alive.

                                                  25 September 2013

Comfort or confined

I sit in my animal enclosure,
Encased in thick glass and behind bright
        shining tubular steel bars.
I cannot remember how I got here.
Was I encouraged to enter to protect
        myself from the outside world?
Did I enter of my own accord to protect
        myself from potential danger?
Or did I decide to trap myself in the belief
    I would protect others from the heartache of potential loss?

I stare out and can see life moving on.
I can see, but not hear or take part.
There is a young couple walking and laughing,
obviously in love and oblivious to those around them,
protected by each other from things that may come.
That was me once, I had a life.

I turn and see a mother and child.
The mother anxious to let go of her child's hand,
yet trying to show her child all the wonders that
        life has to offer.
The child strains to run, to explore.
He breaks free and twirls in the wind, carefree,
        feeling through all his senses.
I was once that child. I was once that mother.
I had a life.

                                              contd...

Next I see a woman.
Clock-watching and walking at pace with shoulders
 hunched and stress etched on her face.
Is she late for work?
Trying to fit in too many daily chores into an
 already over-packed life?
Is she wishing she could be perfect?
A wife.
A mother with all the time to answer questions,
 and the best at her job?
That was me once.
I may have been stressed, but I once had a life.

What now?
I want to take part in life again,
 with all its anxieties, stresses and pleasures.
I want to mix again.
To be that young child, that young person who is carefree.
I want to have a chance to be that anxious mother again.
I even envy the stressed-out woman with no time.
If I could get out, would I change anything?
Would I make different decision to protect myself?

The answer is no.
On the outside it is the ups and downs that create life.

Yet still I sit and gaze out.
Terrified to leave my safe space in case more
 bad things happen to me.
Had my safe house become a cage?
There has always been a key on the inside of the door.
I am free to leave whenever I want and rejoin society.
Yet I sit, scared and removed.
Do I dare to turn the key?

21 Feb 2014

A chance encounter

This week I met a young lady
10 years my junior if not more.
We were standing in the hospital lift.
When everyone else got out, we were heading for floor six.
We both knew what this meant.
The cancer floor, the chemo floor.
The floor for those who face this battle.

This girl was huddled over, in pain and trying to hide it.
We talked as we walked side by side.
Despite her pain she smiled as she spoke.
She had pancreatic cancer, spread to the liver, diagnosed last
                October.
I have lymphoma, diagnosed 2 years ago.

Cancer patients always share this information.
Where is it?
How far along the journey are you?
It's the thing that binds us. The thing we can all understand.

For both a gentle acceptance and acknowledgement
                that life will never be the same again.
We both agreed this is not a bad thing.
We feel privileged to have an altered view on life.
To face death makes you more alive.
It makes you appreciate everything around you and
                helps you focus on what is important to you.

As we separated to go to our own wards,
We shared a hearty good luck.
Neither of us know what the future holds,
But for a brief moment we were allies in our journey.

11 May 2014

Life is just one day

I can choose how I live my life.
I have a choice every minute of every day.
To which situations I react and what form
        that reaction takes.
Choices are mine, and mine alone.

I could choose to live in the past.
To reflect on what could have been.
What would I be doing now
If illness had not been seen.

I could choose to live in the past.
To feel bad for wrongs I have done,
Wishing I could replay my life
Not letting go, holding on.

I could choose to live in the future,
To think of all the things I'll do.
All the times I could spend with others
All the places I could travel to.

I could choose to live in the future,
Dreaming of times yet to come.
While all the world goes on around me
I'll be waiting for my time of fun.

Or I can choose to live for today.
To live each moment as if it is my last.
To spend this, right now, right here.
Not living in the future or past.
Life is made up of just one day

24 hours, more minutes than I dare to know
And I have the choice on how to spend it.
What will today's choices show?

                                      23 Jan 2015

The waiting room

Sitting in a waiting room once again,
Checked in, the man doesn't know my name.
I'm just one of an endless stream of patients,
All painfully ill. All look the same.

I'm called to the blood room.
Routine is under way,
Weigh in and then arm exposed
How many vials will they take today?

They try to make the place look nice
Welcoming comfy chair,
Art on the walls and information on the walls
But to me it feels stark and bare.

Hands start to shake as my wait lengthens
What will today's appointment bring
I dare not hope for any good news
Each time I dare, I'm thrown back into the
        fighting ring.

Trying to calm my breathing.
Trying so hard to relax and chill
Trying to think of anything else
Anything other than the news, news that could
        emotionally kill.

4 Feb 2015

A letter to my doctor

Dear Doctor,

I want you to know how much I appreciate the wonderful work you do. Without you, I would not be alive now. I realise how difficult it must be to juggle so many patients, budgets, and delivering awful news. I am thankful that you strive tirelessly to drive forward research and offer the newest treatments that give the best hope. Thank you for your drive and enthusiasm and commitment.

However, for just one day I would love for you to accompany me on my hospital visit. I'd like you to sit beside me in the waiting room as my friend, and watch as I become more and more anxious as time passes, see me try to distract myself, then lapsing into silence as I worry. I'd like you to try to keep me positive as my friends do during this time. You would notice me flinch each time a doctor walks past or a name is called.

I'd then like you to attend my appointment and be my friend. To listen to the news and how it is delivered. To watch me as I try to keep my chin up and be brave. To know the face I am showing the doctor is a mask, a pretence that I can cope with anything thrown at me and it's all fine. I'd like you to feel with your heart as you hear bad news being delivered and see inside me as a little more of my heart breaks and my resolve threatens to crumble.

I'd then like you to accompany me for the rest of the day as this appointment is only the beginning. Share with me as I phone my parents to tell them the bad news. Hear the stunned disbelief in their voices and see how once again they realise that one day they may have to bury their daughter.

Join in as my husband hold me for dear life and begs me not to give up. Feel the fear he does.

Then sit with me while I sit my children down and tell them the news. They are children! They try so hard to be brave and support me, but at the end of the day they have been through so much that has robbed them of their innocence.

Watch me after I have done this. As I try to be positive for everyone. Note how I am trying not to throw up as the stress takes hold of me physically. See me shake. Sit with me through the night as my mask slips and dark thoughts take hold. Observe the panic attack.

Doctor, I realise you are human and you have to protect yourself. How else could you continue to do your job? How could you be so good at what you do each day? But for one day I'd like you to see the other side. To see how powerfully words affect. To see how a 10-minute appointment has far reaching consequences. And for just one day, just once, to let this into your heart and soul.

Suzanne

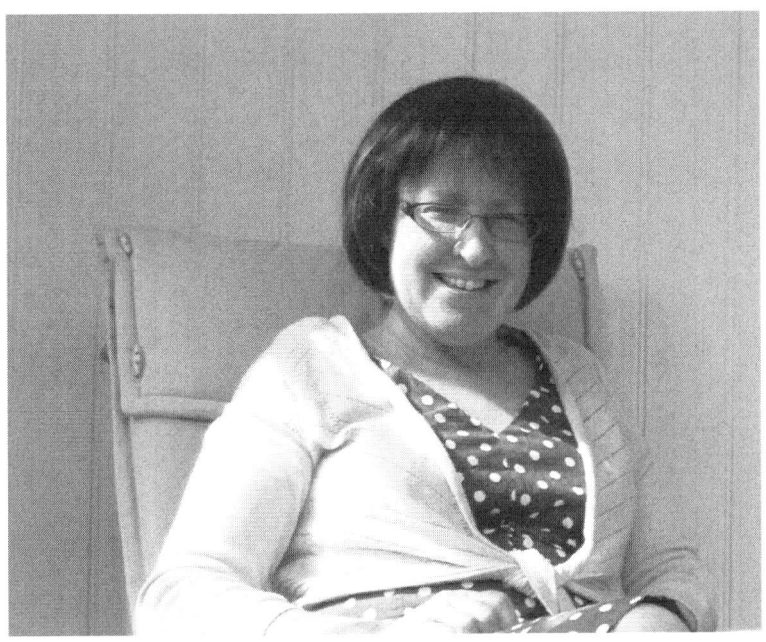

ABOUT SUZANNE CROSSLEY

Suzanne Jane Marshall was born in Lincoln in 1971.

The family moved to Warwickshire in 1973 and she became the proud older sister of Clare, who was born in 1976. She was educated in her early years in Studley and Alcester Grammar school, and was successful in gaining a place at Warwick University. Suzanne passed her four-year BA course with Qualified Teacher Status in 1993 and began her much-loved teaching career in schools in Birmingham and Worcestershire.

She married Andrew Crossley in 1991 and they became the proud parents of two sons, Ben and Matthew. Suzanne continued teaching in Worcestershire until her cancer diagnosis in 2012 when she retired due to ill health.

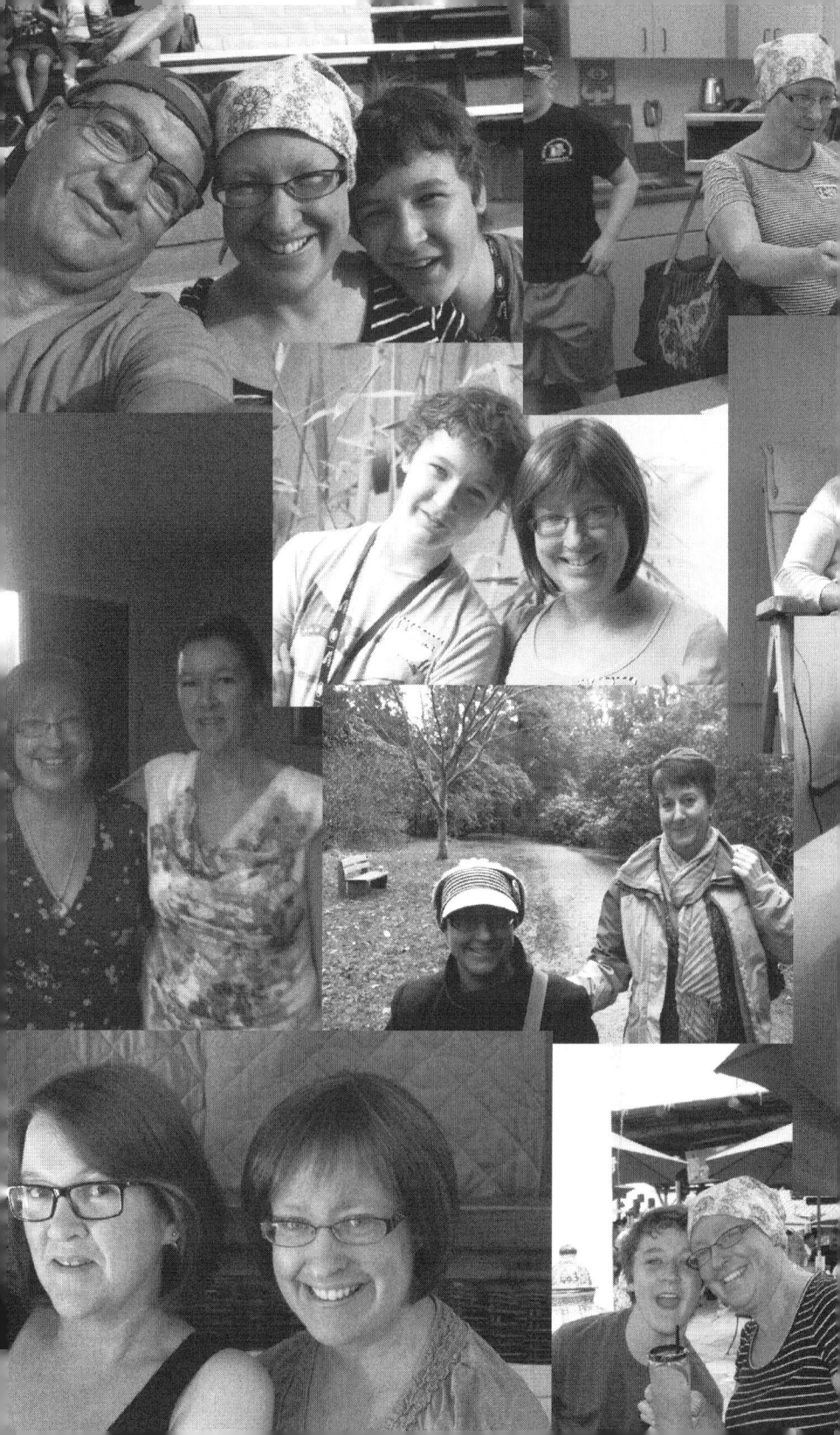

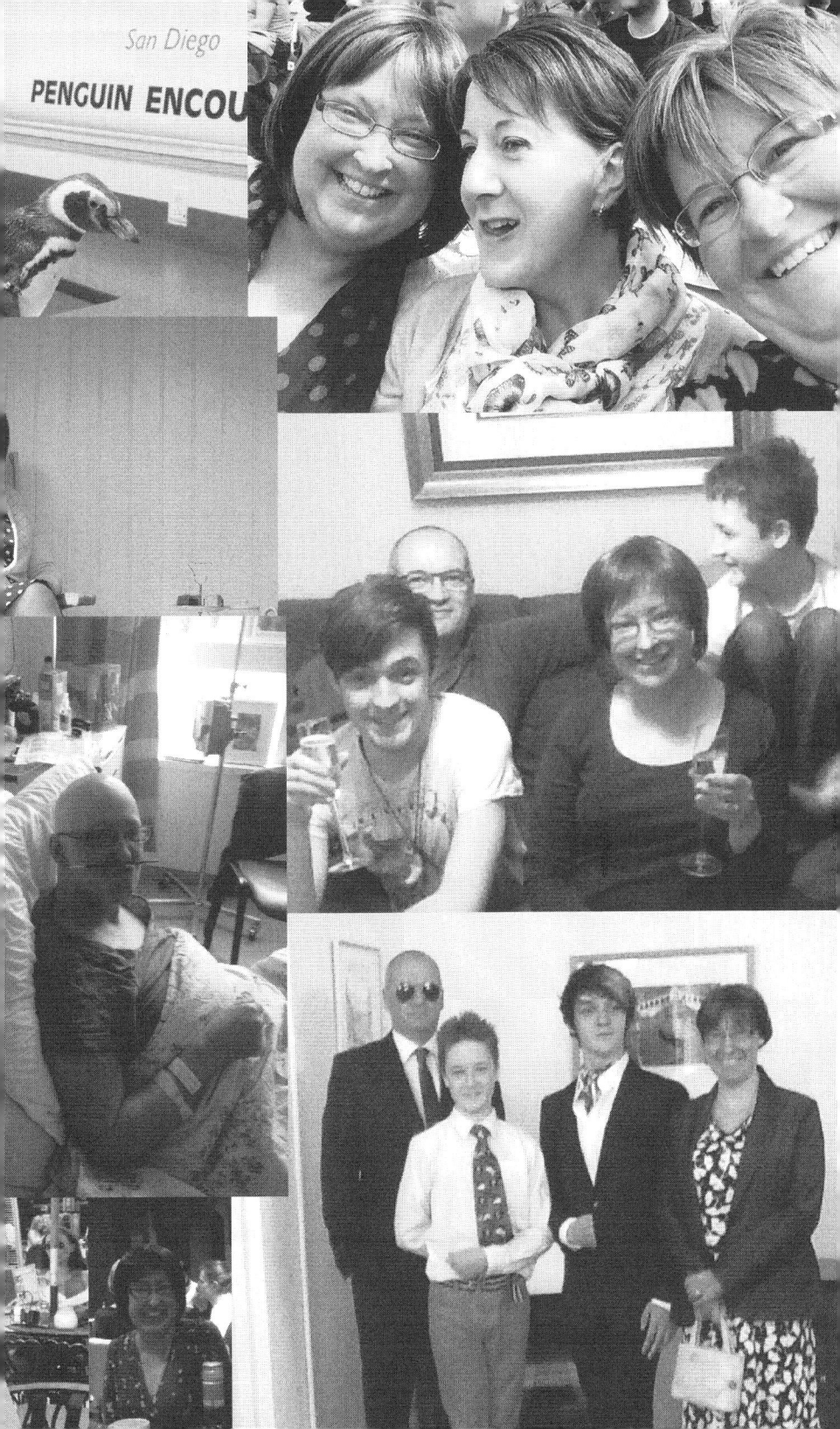

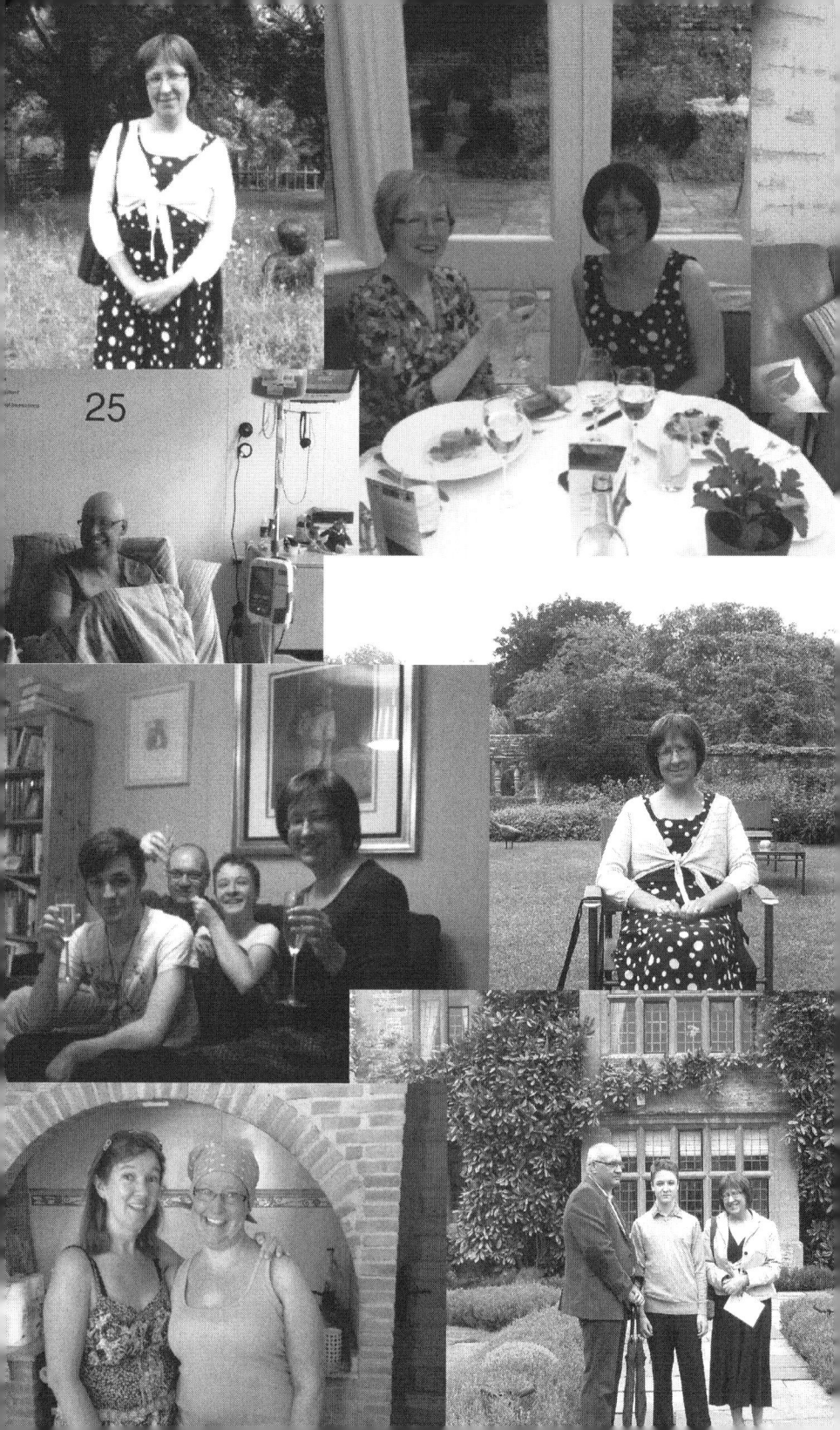

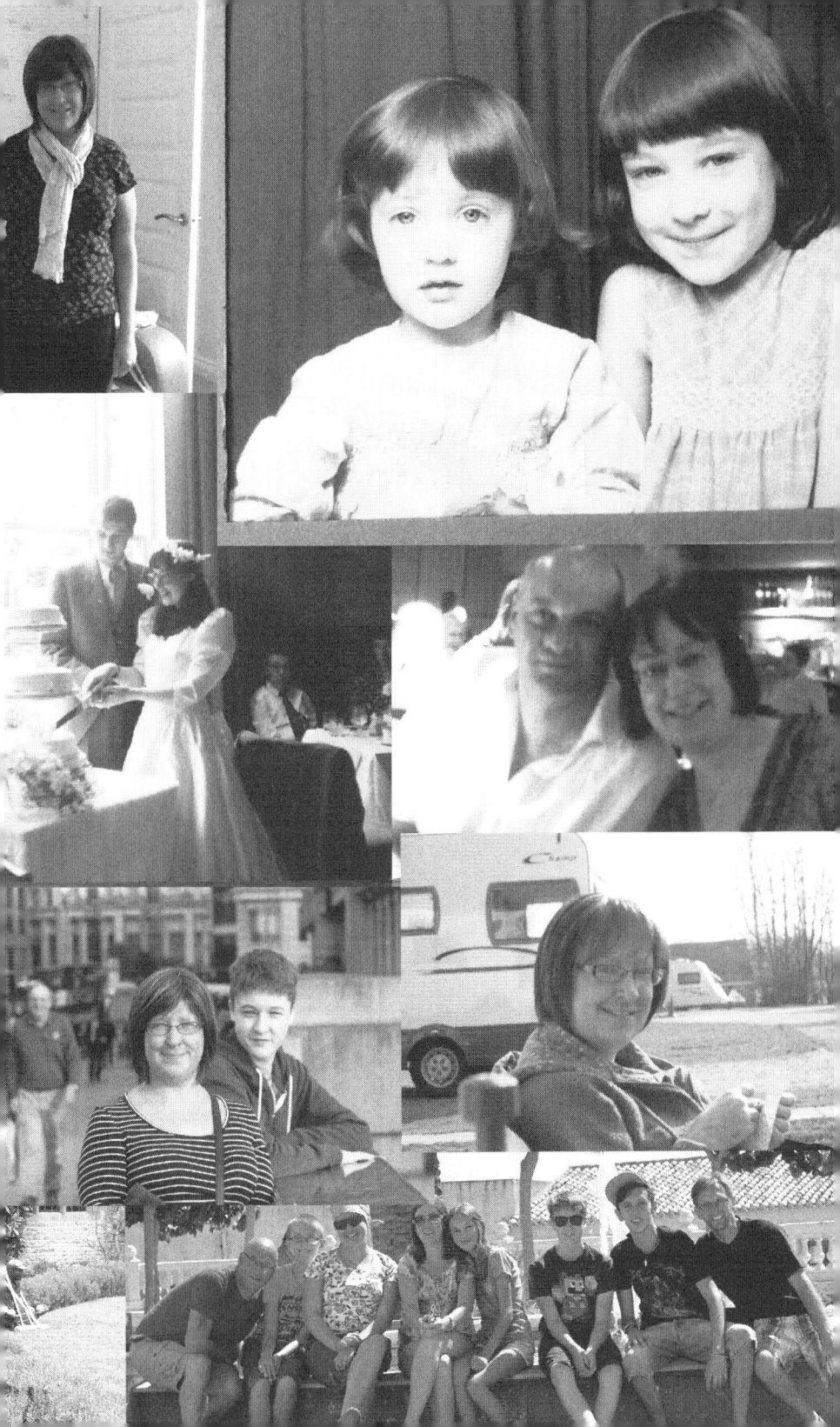

Non Fiction History

Anne Boleyn's Letter from the Tower - **Sandra Vasoli**
Jasper Tudor - **Debra Bayani**
Tudor Places of Great Britain - **Claire Ridgway**
Illustrated Kings and Queens of England - **Claire Ridgway**
A History of the English Monarchy - **Gareth Russell**
The Fall of Anne Boleyn - **Claire Ridgway**
George Boleyn: Tudor Poet, Courtier & Diplomat - **Ridgway & Cherry**
The Anne Boleyn Collection - **Claire Ridgway**
The Anne Boleyn Collection II - **Claire Ridgway**
Two Gentleman Poets at the Court of Henry VIII - **Edmond Bapst**
A Mountain Road - **Douglas Weddell Thompson**

"History in a Nutshell Series"

Sweating Sickness in a Nutshell - **Claire Ridgway**
Mary Boleyn in a Nutshell - **Sarah Bryson**
Thomas Cranmer in a Nutshell - **Beth von Staats**
Henry VIII's Health in a Nutshell - **Kyra Kramer**
Catherine Carey in a Nutshell - **Adrienne Dillard**
The Pyramids in a Nutshell - **Charlotte Booth**

Historical Fiction

Struck with the Dart of Love: Je Anne Boleyn 1 -
The Colour of Poison - **Toni Mount**
Between Two Kings: A Novel of Anne Boleyn - **Olivia Longueville**
Phoenix Rising - **Hunter S. Jones**
Cor Rotto - **Adrienne Dillard**
The Claimant - **Simon Anderson**
The Truth of the Line - **Melanie V. Taylor**

Children's Books

All about Richard III - **Amy Licence**
All about Henry VII - **Amy Licence**
All about Henry VIII - **Amy Licence**
Tudor Tales William at Hampton Court - **Alan Wybrow**

PLEASE LEAVE A REVIEW

If this book was helpful to you, *please* leave a review at the book seller where you purchased it. There is no better way to thank the author's family.
Thank you in advance.

Printed in Great Britain
by Amazon